Kalachakra
and other
Six-Session Yoga Texts

Kalachakra
and other
Six-Session Yoga Texts

translated by
Alexander Berzin

Snow Lion Publications
Ithaca, New York

Snow Lion Publications
P.O. Box 6483
Ithaca, New York 14851 USA
607-273-8519

Printed in Canada on acid-free, recycled paper.

ISBN 1-55939-108-1

Library of Congress Cataloging-in-Publication Data
Kalachakra and other six-session yoga texts / translated by Alexander Berzin
    p.   cm.
    Contents: An extremely abbreviated six-session yoga [Thun-drug-gi rnal-'byor
    mdor-bsdus-pa] / Ngülchu Darma-badra [dNgul-chu Dharmabhadra] -- An
    abbreviated six-session yoga [Thun-drug-gi rnal-'byor bsdus-pa] / by Ngülchu
    Jedrung Lozang-tendzin [dNgul-chu rJe-drung Blo-bzang bstan-'dzin] -- An
    extensive six-session yoga [Thun-drug-gi rnal-'byor rgyas-pa] / by the First
    Panchen Lama [Panchen Blo-bzang chos-kyi rgyal mtshan] and expanded by
    Pabongka [Pha-bong-kha Byams-pa bstan-'dzin 'phrin-las rgya-mtsho] --
    Kalachakra guru-yoga in conjunction with six-session practice [Thun-drug-dang
    'brel-ba'i dus-'khor bla-ma'i rnal-'byor dpag-bsam yongs-'du'i snye-ma] by the
    Fourteenth Dalai Lama [bsTan-'dzin rgya-mtsho] and versified by Yongdzin
    Ling Rinpochey [Yongs-'dzin gLing Thub-bstan lung-rtogs rnam-rgyal 'phrin-
    las].
    ISBN 1-55939-108-1 (alk. paper)
    1. Kālacakra (Tantric rite)--China--Tibet--Early works to 1800. 2. Yoga (Tantric
Buddhism)--Early works to 1800. I. Berzin, Alexander.
BQ7699.K34K356 1998
294.3'438--dc21   98-17366
                                                                              CIP

Table of Contents

An Extremely Abbreviated Six-Session Yoga

(Thun-drug-gi rnal-'byor mdor-bsdus-pa)

by

Ngülchu Darma-badra
(dNgul-chu Dharmabhadra)

An Extremely Abbreviated
Six-Session Yoga

From my gurus and the Three Precious Gems,
    I take safe direction.
With myself clear as a deity, holding vajra and bell,
    I present you with offerings.
Upholding the teachings of sutra and tantra, I restrain
    myself from a wide array of faulty deeds.
Amassing within all constructive measures, I benefit
    beings through the four types of giving.

An Abbreviated Six-Session Yoga

(Thun-drug-gi rnal-'byor bsdus-pa)

by

Ngülchu Jedrung Lozang-tendzin

(dNgul-chu rJe-drung Blo-bzang bstan-'dzin)

An Abbreviated Six-Session Yoga

From my heart, I take safe direction from the Three Precious Gems.
May I free all beings from torment and place them in everlasting bliss.
To become fully enlightened for their sake, I develop bodhichitta
And train myself through bodhisattva acts.

In the sky before me, on a throne, a lotus, a sun and moon,
Sits my root guru, the all-pervading master, Vajradhara,
With blue-colored body, holding vajra and bell,
Embracing Dhatu-ishvari and sporting with co-arising bliss.

Three spots on your body are marked with three letters.
Light radiates forth from the *HUM* at your heart,
Inviting here beings for deep awareness:
You become of one taste.

At your lotus feet I bow, Vajradhara, and present you with
An ocean of clouds of outer, inner and hidden offerings.
Mount Meru, the continents, a jeweled treasure vase,
    the sun and the moon:
These peerless offerings of Samanta-bhadra, I make unto you.

Every supreme and mundane attainment
Follows upon pure devotion to you, my spiritual guide.
Seeing this, I forsake my body and even my life,
Inspire me to practice what only will please you.

Requested like this, my guru alights on the crown of my head.
We merge, becoming inseparably one taste.
Now I, Vajrasattva, holding vajra and bell, embracing Bhagavati,
Sport with co-arising blissful awareness.
With no sense of a loss, I donate my land, my body and wealth,
    and all virtues amassed throughout the three times
In order to help all mothers.
I shall never transgress, though my life be at stake,
    the limits of the precepts
Of my pratimoksha, bodhisattva or tantric vows.

Upholding the scriptural and realized Dharma
Gathered in three sutra vehicles and four tantra sets,
I shall liberate beings with their skillful means.

I dedicate this virtue so that the deeds and prayers
Of the Buddhas and bodhisattvas may all be fulfilled
And the hallowed Dharma be upheld.

By inspiration from the supreme Triple Gem
And the force of infallible dependent arising,
May all my wonderful prayers come true
And I quickly attain the state of a Buddha.

An Extensive Six-Session Yoga

(Thun-drug-gi rnal-'byor rgyas-pa)

by

the First Panchen Lama

(Paṇ-chen Blo-bzang chos-kyi rgyal-mtshan)

and expanded by

Pabongka

(Pha-bong-kha Byams-pa bstan-'dzin 'phrin-las rgya-mtsho)

An Extensive Six-Session Yoga

[A1]

I take safe direction, until enlightened,
From the Buddhas, the Dharma and the Highest Assembly.
By the positive force of my giving and so on,
May I become a Buddha to benefit all.
[*3x, only for the first repetition*]

May all beings be parted from clinging and aversion —
    feeling close to some and distant from others.
May they win the bliss that is specially sublime.
May they find release from the sea of unbearable sorrow.
May they never be parted from freedom's true joy.

From this moment on, until I'm a Buddha,
I shall never give up, though my life be at stake,
The attitude wishing to gain full enlightenment
In order to free from the fears of samsara
And nirvana's complacency all sentient beings.

O Buddhas, bodhisattvas and gurus please listen.
Just as past Buddhas have developed bodhichitta,
Then trained by stages through bodhisattva acts,
I likewise develop bodhichitta to benefit beings
And train by stages through bodhisattva acts.
[*3x, only for the first repetition*]

Now my life has become truly fruitful,
For having attained a human existence
Today I've been born in the family of Buddhas
And now have become Buddha's spiritual child.

Now in whatever way possible
I shall act in accord with this family,
Never causing disgrace
To this noble clan that lacks any fault.

[A-X]

In the sky before me, on a breath-taking throne of jewels,
On top of an opened lotus and symbolic discs of a sun and moon,
Sits my root guru, the all-pervading master, Vajradhara,
With a blue-colored body, one face and two arms,
Holding vajra and bell, and embracing a motherly likeness.
Shining resplendent with the major and minor marks of a Buddha,
Adorned with lavish jeweled ornaments,
Draped with fine garments of enchanting, heavenly scarves —
The mere thought of you quenches all my torment.
With a nature encompassing every superlative
    source of direction,
You sit cross-legged in the vajra position,
Three spots on your body marked with three letters.
Light radiates from the *HUM* at your heart,
Inviting Guru Vajradhara from his natural abode.
JAH HUM BAM HO, you become non-dual.

[A2]

I bow at your lotus-feet,
O my jewel-like Guru Vajradhara,
Your kindness heralds
An instantaneous dawn of great bliss.

[A-X]

OM — I bow to you, Bhagavan, Lord of the Brave Ones —
HUM HUM PHAT
OM — To you with brilliance equaling the fire that ends a great eon —
HUM HUM PHAT
OM — To you with a crown of dread locks —
HUM HUM PHAT
OM — To you with bared fangs and a fearsome face —
HUM HUM PHAT
OM — To you with myriad arms blazing with light —
HUM HUM PHAT
OM — To you wielding an axe, an uplifted lasso, a spear and skull-staff —
HUM HUM PHAT
OM — To you wearing a tiger-skin wrap —
HUM HUM PHAT
OM — I bow to you with a magnificent smoke-colored body that ends
all obstruction — *HUM HUM PHAT*

OM — I bow to you, Bhagavati, Vajra-varahi —
HUM HUM PHAT
OM — To you, noble queen of awareness, invincible throughout the
three realms — *HUM HUM PHAT*
OM — To you destroying all fears of elemental spirits with your great
vajra — *HUM HUM PHAT*
OM — To you sitting on your vajra-seat, invincible to others, with eyes
that mesmerize — *HUM HUM PHAT*
OM — To you with a fearsome body of fiery tummo desiccating
Brahma — *HUM HUM PHAT*

OM — To you victorious over opposing forces, terrifying and drying
  up demons — *HUM HUM PHAT*
OM — To you who triumph over all that can make you bewildered,
  dumbfounded or stupefied — *HUM HUM PHAT*
OM — I bow to you, Vajra-varahi, yogini, queen of desire —
  HUM HUM PHAT

[A3]

All things I possess and what is not mine,
What I actually arrange or create from my mind —
I present you with an ocean of clouds of various offerings:
Outer, inner and enigmatic.

The body, speech and mind of myself and others,
Whatever we enjoy as well as our bountiful store
Of constructive potential from throughout the three times,
A splendid jeweled mandala and expansive Samanta-bhadra offerings —
I envision these all and present them to you,
O my guru, my yidam, my Three Precious Gems.
Accepting them out of the force of compassion,
Grant me inspiring strength.
IDAM GURU RATNA MANDALAKAM NIRYATA-YAMI.

I humbly beseech you, my precious guru,
Just as the Buddhas of all times and directions have tamed what needs be,
You likewise enact Buddha-deeds in countless realms
Sporting the guise of a monk clad in saffron.

I humbly beseech you, my precious guru,
Esteemed by Vajradhara, for those of dim mind,
As a field of merit more holy than
The endless circles of infinite Buddhas.

Every supreme and mundane attainment
Follows upon pure devotion to you, my spiritual guide.
Seeing this I forsake my body and even my life,
Inspire me to practice what only will please you.

[B-X]

Requested like this, my supreme guru
Alights on the crown of my head.

[B1]

Gladly merging once more with me,
We become of one taste.

With the pride of Vajrasattva, holding vajra and bell,
Symbolic of the hidden factors of co-arising great bliss
And the state by nature fantasy-free,
I embrace Bhagavati.

From this moment on, with no sense of a loss,
I donate my body, and likewise my wealth,
And my virtues amassed throughout the three times
In order to help all beings, my mothers.

[B-X]

Praising myself and belittling others,
Not sharing Dharma teachings or wealth,
Not listening even if others apologize,
Discarding mahayana teachings,
Stealing goods belonging to the Triple Gem,
Forsaking the Dharma,
Stealing from those clad in saffron,
Committing any of the five heinous crimes,
Holding a distorted, antagonistic outlook,
Destroying places such as towns,
Teaching voidness to those whose minds are untrained,
Turning others' aim away from enlightenment,
Causing others to discard their pratimoksha vows,
Belittling the shravaka teachings,
Proclaiming a false realization of what is profound,
Accepting goods belonging to the Triple Gem,

Establishing unfair policies,
Giving up bodhichitta —
These are the eighteen root downfalls from the bodhisattva vows;
I shall safeguard against them.

Not regarding them as detrimental,
Not forsaking the wish to repeat such acts,
Delighting and taking pleasure in them,
And having no sense of honor or face
Are the four binding factors that must all be present
For sixteen of these to be complete.
For either a distorted outlook or giving up bodhichitta,
These four are not needed.

Scorning or deriding my guru,
Disregarding any ethical training,
Faulting my vajra brothers or sisters,
Abandoning love for any being,
Giving up aspiring or engaged bodhichitta,
Deriding the teachings of sutra or tantra,
Revealing confidential teachings to those unripe,
Reviling my aggregates,
Rejecting voidness,
Being loving toward malevolent people,
Not maintaining continual mindfulness of a correct view,
Deterring those with faith,
Not properly relying on closely bonding materials,
Deriding women —
These are the fourteen root tantric downfalls;
I shall safeguard against them at the cost of my life.

Forsaking the four root destructive actions, likewise liquor and
    faulty behavior,
Committing myself whole-heartedly to a holy protecting guru,
Serving and treating respectfully Dharma friends,
Cultivating the ten constructive acts,

Avoiding the causes for forsaking mahayana,
Belittling it or treading on objects worthy of respect —
I shall honor these further practices to bond me closely.

Relying on an unqualified mudra partner,
Sitting in union devoid of the three recognitions,
Showing confidential objects to an unsuitable vessel,
Fighting or arguing when offering tsog,
Giving false answers to sincerely asked questions,
Staying more than a week in a shravaka's home,
Boasting that I am a yogi, although I am not,
Teaching the sacred Dharma to those with no faith,
Improperly engaging in mandala-rites, such as without a retreat,
Transgressing pratimoksha or bodhisattva trainings
    when there is no need,
Acting counter to the teachings of *Fifty Stanzas on the Guru* —
These are the secondary tantric heavy actions;
I shall safeguard against them in accord with the rules.

I shall not look down on left-handed behavior,
I shall offer tsog, reject sitting in union with an
    unqualified partner,
While in union, never be parted from a correct view,
Relentlessly aspire to the path of desire,
Not forsake the two kinds of mudra,
Exert effort mainly on the outer and inner methods,
Never release my subtle jasmine drops,
Commit myself to chaste behavior,
And abandon nausea when imbibing bodhichitta.

[B2]

I shall never transgress, even in dreams,
The most minor rule of the pure moral trainings
Of the pratimoksha, bodhisattva or tantric vows.
I shall practice according to Buddha's words.

As Buddha intended, I shall uphold the complete sacred Dharma
Of the scriptures and realizations gathered in
The three sutra vehicles and four tantra sets.
I shall liberate all beings by means that suit each.

[C1]

Through the force of the positive potential derived from this
And the power of Vajradhara, may I never transgress,
Throughout all my lives, the limits of my precepts.
May I complete the stages of the twofold path.

In brief, may I be born in Shambhala, the storehouse of gems,
And in as quick a time as the amount of ennobling,
Constructive potential I have gathered, for example by this,
Complete there the stages of this peerless path.

May I make full use of the glory of Dharma, never being bereft
Of perfect gurus throughout all my lives,
And by achieving in full the talents of all the stages and paths,
May I quickly attain Vajradhara-enlightenment.

———————◆•◆———————

If reciting six times each day in the manner of three times each morning
and three times each evening, recite the following sequence:

- [A] three times, omitting all [A-X] sections for the second and
  third repetitions,
- [B] three times, omitting all [B-X] sections for the second and
  third repetitions,
- [C] one time.

Kalachakra Guru-Yoga
in Conjunction with Six-Session Practice:

A Cluster of Fruit from an
All-Embracing Wish-Granting Tree

(Thun-drug-dang 'brel-ba'i dus-'khor bla-ma'i rnal-'byor
dpag-bsam yongs-'du'i snye-ma)

by
the Fourteenth Dalai Lama
(rGyal-dbang bsTan-'dzin rgya-mtsho)

and versified by
Yongdzin Ling Rinpochey
(Yongs-'dzin gLing Thub-bstan lung-rtogs rnam-rgyal 'phrin-las)

Kalachakra Guru-Yoga
in Conjunction with Six-Session Practice

[A1]

From the Buddhas and my foremost empowering master,
The Dharma of uncleavable method and wisdom they show,
And both Sangha divisions abiding in it,
I pure-heartedly take safe direction.
From this moment on, until I'm enlightened,
I dedicate my heart with bodhichitta,
Heighten my resolve and rid myself of
Conceiving of "me" or "myself, the possessor."
[*3x, only for the first repetition*]

I shall meditate now that all beings
Be endowed with happiness,
Parted from grief,
Have the joy of remaining always blissfully aware,
And equanimity toward everyone as equal.
[*3x, only for the first repetition*]

From this moment on, until I'm a Buddha,
I shall never give up, though my life be at stake,
The attitude wishing to gain full enlightenment
In order to free from the fears of samsara
And nirvana's complacency all sentient beings.

O Buddhas, bodhisattvas and gurus please listen.
Just as past Buddhas have developed bodhichitta,
Then trained by stages through bodhisattva acts,
I likewise develop bodhichitta to benefit beings
And train by stages through bodhisattva acts.
[*3x, only for the first repetition*]

Now my life has become truly fruitful,
For having attained a human existence
Today I've been born in the family of Buddhas
And now have become Buddha's spiritual child.

Now in whatever way possible
I shall act in accord with this family,
Never causing disgrace
To this noble clan that lacks any fault.

[A-X]

Within a state of fantasy-free clear light mahamudra,
On the broad path before me of the immortal divines,
Like a glittering multi-colored display of rainbows,
In the center of a billowing ocean of clouds of Samanta-bhadra offerings,
On a throne of jewels held aloft by eight breath-taking lions,
On the face of an opened thousand-petalled lotus delighting the mind,
On top of symbolic discs of a moon, a sun, and Rahu and Kalagni planets,
As a total amalgam into one of as many infinite masses
Of sources of safe direction as there are,
Inseparable from my kind guru,
Stands the magnificent Bhagavan, Kalachakra,
Imbued with the lustrous hue of a sapphire, blazing with brilliance,
With one face and two arms, holding vajra and bell.

To symbolize the uncommon path
Of unity of method and wisdom,
Your manner of appearance is being in union

With Vishva-mata, saffron in color,
Holding a cleaver and skullcup.

With your right leg red and outstretched,
Your left one white and bent,
Dancing on top of a Mara and Rudra,
You are elegant with hundreds of artistic tones.

Your body, adorned with jewelry inspiring awe,
Like the vault of the heavens
Beautifully studded with clusters of stars,
Stands amidst an effulgence
Of five-colored stainless light,
Exuding joy, with three bodily points
In the nature of three vajra-deities
Taking the form of letters begotten of light.

Emanated from the seed-syllable at your heart,
Vajra-vega, holding a bevy of fearsome weapons,
Hooks in firmly a host of sources of direction,
Living in infinite pure-land abodes,
To become of an equal taste
With you who are here to bond me closely.
You now assume the grand nature of being
An amalgam of every safe source of direction.

[A2]

Respectfully I prostrate to you,
My guru with a trio of inseparable bodies:
A dharma-kaya of greatly blissful awareness,
Primordially fantasy-free;
A sambhoga-kaya possessing five,
The reflexive appearance of your deep awareness;
And a nirmana-kaya of enlightening dancers,
Emanated throughout the ocean of the wanderers' sphere.

[A-X]

OM — I bow to you, Bhagavan, Lord of the Brave Ones —
  HUM HUM PHAT
OM — To you with brilliance equaling the fire that ends a great eon —
  HUM HUM PHAT
OM — To you with a crown of dread locks —
  HUM HUM PHAT
OM — To you with bared fangs and a fearsome face —
  HUM HUM PHAT
OM — To you with myriad arms blazing with light —
  HUM HUM PHAT
OM — To you wielding an axe, an uplifted lasso, a spear and skull-staff —
  HUM HUM PHAT
OM — To you wearing a tiger-skin wrap —
  HUM HUM PHAT
OM — I bow to you with a magnificent smoke-colored body that ends
  all obstruction — *HUM HUM PHAT*

OM — I bow to you, Bhagavati, Vajra-varahi —
  HUM HUM PHAT
OM — To you, noble queen of awareness, invincible throughout the
  three realms — *HUM HUM PHAT*
OM — To you destroying all fears of elemental spirits with your great
  vajra — *HUM HUM PHAT*
OM — To you sitting on your vajra-seat, invincible to others, with eyes
  that mesmerize — *HUM HUM PHAT*
OM — To you with a fearsome body of fiery tummo desiccating
  Brahma — *HUM HUM PHAT*
OM — To you victorious over opposing forces, terrifying and drying
  up demons — *HUM HUM PHAT*
OM — To you who triumph over all that can make you bewildered,
  dumbfounded or stupefied — *HUM HUM PHAT*
OM — I bow to you, Vajra-varahi, yogini, queen of desire —
  HUM HUM PHAT

[A3]

Billowing masses of clouds of offerings,
Outer, inner and enigmatic,
Both actually arrayed and created
From the play of my absorbed concentration,
And six pair of slender-bodied, delightful bestowers of bliss
With lotus-hands stunningly beautiful with gifts worthy to offer —
Such common and uncommon presents as these,
As well as my body, whatever I enjoy
And the bountiful store of my constructive potential,
I offer to you, with a mind unattached,
Undaunted and clear about the three circles involved,
O my bountiful field, my kind sublime guru,
That I might please you.

The body, speech and mind of myself and others,
Whatever we enjoy, as well as our bountiful store
Of constructive potential from throughout the three times,
A splendid jeweled mandala and expansive Samanta-bhadra offerings --
I envision these all and present them to you,
O my guru, my yidam, my Three Precious Gems.
Accepting them out of the force of compassion,
Grant me inspiring strength.
IDAM GURU RATNA MANDALAKAM NIRYATA-YAMI.

Every negative act and downfall I've made or caused others
    to commit
Due to the stallion of my mind, wild and untamed from
    beginningless time,
Being drunk with the spirits of the reckless three emotions of poison,
And especially my actions breaking my bonds
With the general and specific traits of the five Buddha families —
Such as disturbing my guru's mind or breaching his words —
Also my not safeguarding correctly the twenty-five types

Of tamed behavior and so forth,
Whatever disgraceful actions I've done, I openly admit,
With a strong mind of regret and the promise to restrain
From doing them again.

I rejoice in the ocean of my own and others' well-done deeds
Producing a bounteous foam of delightful results.
I request you to let a monsoonal rain fall of three vehicles of Dharma
Suiting the thoughts and tempers of modest, middling
And supreme disciples needing to be tamed.
With a body of coarse forms that can appear to the face
Of those who look from this side of omniscience,
Please remain here without dissipation,
Unchanging and stable for hundreds of eons.
I dedicate my bountiful store of constructive potential,
For example from this,
As a cause for my quickly attaining
The unity of enlightenment as a Kalachakra.

[A-X]

From this moment on, until I'm enlightened,
I dedicate my heart with bodhichitta,
Heighten my resolve and rid myself of
Conceiving of "me" or "myself, the possessor."

I shall actualize, for the sake of the three bountiful stores,
The far-reaching attitudes of giving, ethical discipline,
Tolerance, enthusiasm, constancy of mind,
Discriminating awareness, skill in means,
Aspiration, strength and deep awareness.

I shall meditate now that all beings
Be endowed with happiness,
Parted from grief,
Have the joy of remaining always blissfully aware,
And equanimity toward everyone as equal.

I shall hail them with a wave of giving
And, having spoken with pleasing words,
Cheer them with meaningful behavior
And implant them with eminent advice
By acting accordingly.

I shall rid myself of the ten destructive acts:
Three physical actions, four kinds of speech,
And three ways of thinking.

I shall remove the five obstacles:
Regret, foggy-mindedness,
Sleepiness, flightiness of mind,
And indecisive wavering —
They hinder my three higher trainings.

I shall rid myself of attachment, hostility,
Foolish ignorance and pride:
The four emotions that disturb me,
Anchoring the root of my compulsive existence.

I shall depose the confusion of my sensory desires,
Compulsive existence, lack of awareness,
And outlook on life: the four forms of confusion
Causing my uncontrollably recurring existence.

A total absence, lack of a sign,
Lack of a hope and lack of an action to affect things ahead:
Through these four gateways to full liberation,
I shall actualize total enlightenment.

[A4]

O kind Guru, amalgam of the Triple Gem,
When I commit you my heart, you're a wish-granting source
Spouting the milk of all positive aims
For compulsive existence or serene liberation.
I request you bestow on my mind-stream inspiring strength.

OM AH GURU VAJRA-DHARA, VAGINDRA SUMATI, SHASANA
    DHARA, SAMUDRA SHRI BHADRA, SARVA SIDDHI HUM HUM
[*repeat as many times as possible*]

[A-X]

I request you, Guru Kalachakra,
Confer on me fully all the empowerments,
Inspire me to cleanse obscuration from my four family traits
And thus to achieve a Buddha's four bodies. [3x]

Empowering deities emanated from your heart,
Together with the male and female Buddhas
And their surrounding figures from your mandala palace,
Confer the water, crown, ear tassel, vajra and bell,
Tamed behavior, name and subsequent permission empowerments,
And then supremely confer the two sets
Of higher and highest four empowerments
And the empowerments of a vajra master.

By means of these, the energy-channels and winds of my body
Become flexible and fit.
Empowered to meditate on both stages of practice,
I gain the good fortune to fully deplete
The twenty-one thousand six hundred winds of my karma
Plus every bit of my body's corporeal matter,
And thus to manifest in this very lifetime
Kalachakra-enlightenment endowed sevenfold.

[B-X]

Having made my requests with respect from my heart
To you, my guru, O great Vajradhara,
Master amalgamating infinite sources of safe direction,
I request you bestow on my mind-stream inspiring strength.

[B1]

By the force of request,
Through my strong plaintive yearning,
My root guru, great Kalachakra,
Alights on the crown of my head.

Gladly merging with me,
We become of one taste.
All phenomena — causes, effects, natures and actions —
Like an illusion or dream, are, from the start,
Utterly devoid of solid reality.

Within a state of this absence, like a surfacing bubble,
Comes a water-born lotus with petals outspread.
On its corolla are stacked symbolic discs
Of a moon, a sun, Rahu and Kalagni.

On top of them, in the nature of my white and red sources,
Are a moon and a sun, their perimeters embellished
With garlands of vowels and consonants
In the nature of the major and minor marks of a Buddha,
And their center embedded with syllables *HUM* and *HI*,
Symbolizing my energy-wind and mind.

These mix into one in the form of a syllable *HAM*
From which I transform and arise, Kalachakra,
Imbued with the lustrous hue of a sapphire, blazing with brilliance,
Having four faces and twenty-four arms.

To symbolize the vajra of supreme, unchanging blissful awareness
And the actual state devoid of all fantasized ways of existing,
My first two hands hold a vajra and bell,
While embracing my motherly partner.

[B-X]

My remaining lotus-hands on the right and the left
Are arrayed with insignia
Such as cleaver and shield.
My right leg is red and outstretched,
My left one white and bent:
Dancing on top of a Mara and Rudra,
I am elegant with hundreds of artistic tones.

My body, adorned with copious jewelry,
Like the vault of the heavens
Beautifully studded with clusters of stars,
Stands amidst an effulgence
Of five-colored stainless light.

Facing me, the Bhagavan, is Vishva-mata,
Saffron in color, four faces, eight arms,
Holding a variety of insignia
Such as cleaver and skull-cup,
With her left leg outstretched,
And embracing me, the Bhagavan.
We are encircled, in the cardinal and intermediate directions,
By eight shakti maidens
On petals the number of the auspicious signs.

Standing magnificently like this, as the principal figure,
I emanate from my heart a Vajra-vega,
Holding a bevy of fearsome weapons with which
He hooks in firmly a host of sources of direction,
Living in infinite pure-land abodes,
To become of an equal taste
With those I visualize to bond me closely.

Empowering deities confer the empowerments.
As the principal one, along with my circle,
We all become sealed
With the ruling figures of our Buddha families.

The perimeters around the seed-syllables at the hearts
Of myself, the principal figure, along with my circle,
Are ringed with a garland of each of our mantras.
From these emanate a host of mandala deities
Who fulfill the aims of wandering beings
And then gather back, dissolving into the seed-syllables at our hearts.

OM AH HUM HO HKSHMLVRYAM HUM PHAT
[*"HKSHMLVRYAM"* is pronounced in Tibetan *"HANKYA MALA*
   WARAYA," "PHAT" is pronounced *"PAY."*]
OM PHREM VISHVA-MATA HUM HUM PHAT
OM DANA PARAMITA HUM HUM PHAT
OM SHILA PARAMITA HUM HUM PHAT
OM KSHANTI PARAMITA HUM HUM PHAT
OM VIRYA PARAMITA HUM HUM PHAT
OM DHYANA PARAMITA HUM HUM PHAT
OM PRAJNA PARAMITA HUM HUM PHAT
OM UPAYA PARAMITA HUM HUM PHAT
OM PRANIDHANA PARAMITA HUM HUM PHAT
OM BALA PARAMITA HUM HUM PHAT
OM JNANA PARAMITA HUM HUM PHAT
[*repeat these mantras as much as possible*]

OM VAJRA-SATTVA SAMAYA MANU-PALAYA, VAJRA-SATTVA
   TVENO-PATISHTA, DRIDHO ME BHAVA, SU TOSHYO ME BHAVA,
   SU POSHYO ME BHAVA, ANU RAKTO ME BHAVA, SARVA
   SIDDHIM ME PRAYACCHA, SARVA KARMA SUCHA ME,
   CHITTAM SHRIYAM KURU HUM, HA HA HA HA HOH
   BHAGAVAN, SARVA TATHAGATA VAJRA, MA ME MUNCHA,
   VAJRA BHAVA, MAHA SAMAYA SATTVA, AH HUM PHAT

Divine offering maidens emanated from my heart present us the offerings:
OM SHRI KALACHAKRA SAPARI-VARA ARGHAM PRATICCHA
   NAMAH
OM SHRI KALACHAKRA SAPARI-VARA PADYAM PRATICCHA
   NAMAH
OM SHRI KALACHAKRA SAPARI-VARA PROKSHANAM PRATICCHA
   NAMAH

OM SHRI KALACHAKRA SAPARI-VARA ANCHAMANAM PRATICCHA
   NAMAH
OM SHRI KALACHAKRA SAPARI-VARA GANDHAM PRATICCHA
   NAMAH
OM SHRI KALACHAKRA SAPARI-VARA PUSHPE PRATICCHA
   NAMAH
OM SHRI KALACHAKRA SAPARI-VARA DHUPE PRATICCHA
   NAMAH
OM SHRI KALACHAKRA SAPARI-VARA ALOKE PRATICCHA
   NAMAH
OM SHRI KALACHAKRA SAPARI-VARA GANDHE PRATICCHA
   NAMAH
OM SHRI KALACHAKRA SAPARI-VARA NAIVIDYA PRATICCHA
   NAMAH
OM SHRI KALACHAKRA SAPARI-VARA SHABDA PRATICCHA
   NAMAH
OM SHRI KALACHAKRA MANDALAM SAPARI-VARIBHYAH
   NAMAH

I prostrate to you, O glorious Kalachakra.
With a nature of voidness and compassion,
You neither take birth in the three planes of existence,
Nor perish away. Your enlightening bodies,
As a way of knowing and what is known,
Possess the same source.

I bow to you, Kalachakra.
Having rid yourself of unions of vowels with consonants,
And those with the syllables *HUM* and *PHAT*,
You've an enlightening body born from what is unchanging.

I bow to you, O Lady Mahamudra.
You possess the supreme of all aspects
Having the nature of a magic-mirror image,
Beyond an actual nature of atoms.

I prostrate to you, Vishva-mata,
Lady giving birth to all the Buddhas.
Having rid yourself of arising and passing,
You possess the behavior of Samanta-bhadra.

The shakti maidens, as well as our seats,
Melt into light and dissolve into me.
I, as well, melt into light.
Within a non-objectified state of voidness,
I arise once more as a Kalachakra, with one face and two arms.

[B-2]

From this moment on, with no sense of a loss,
I donate my body, and likewise my wealth,
And my virtues amassed throughout the three times
In order to help all beings, my mothers.

[B-X]

Praising myself and belittling others,
Not sharing Dharma teachings or wealth,
Not listening even if others apologize,
Discarding mahayana teachings,
Stealing goods belonging to the Triple Gem,
Forsaking the Dharma,
Stealing from those clad in saffron,
Committing any of the five heinous crimes,
Holding a distorted, antagonistic outlook,
Destroying places such as towns,
Teaching voidness to those whose minds are untrained,
Turning others' aim away from enlightenment,
Causing others to discard their pratimoksha vows,
Belittling the shravaka teachings,
Proclaiming a false realization of what is profound,

Accepting goods belonging to the Triple Gem,
Establishing unfair policies,
Giving up bodhichitta —
These are the eighteen root downfalls from the bodhisattva vows;
I shall safeguard against them.

Not regarding them as detrimental,
Not forsaking the wish to repeat such acts,
Delighting and taking pleasure in them,
And having no sense of honor or face
Are the four binding factors that must all be present
For sixteen of these to be complete.
For either a distorted outlook or giving up bodhicitta,
These four are not needed.

Scorning or deriding my guru,
Disregarding any ethical training,
Faulting my vajra brothers or sisters,
Abandoning love for any being,
Giving up aspiring or engaged bodhichitta,
Deriding the teachings of sutra or tantra,
Revealing confidential teachings to those unripe,
Reviling my aggregates,
Rejecting voidness,
Being loving toward malevolent people,
Not maintaining continual mindfulness of a correct view,
Deterring those with faith,
Not properly relying on closely bonding materials,
Deriding women —
These are the fourteen root tantric downfalls;
I shall safeguard against them at the cost of my life.

Disturbing my guru's mind,
Breaching what he has said,
Emitting my subtle seminal drops,
Holding voidness in sutra or tantra as better or worse and belittling either,
Harboring deceitful love,

Rejecting unchanging blissful awareness,
Faulting yogis —
These constitute the kalachakra root downfalls.

The five destructive actions:
Damaging a life, speaking lies,
Taking what was not given to me,
Indulging in inappropriate sexual behavior,
And drinking alcohol;
The five auxiliary destructive actions:
Gambling, shooting dice or playing board games,
Eating unseemly meat,
Saying whatever comes to mind,
Setting out offerings for ancestor worship,
And sacrificing livestock to make a blood offering;
The five types of murder:
Killing cattle, children, women, men,
And destroying symbols of a Buddha's body, speech or mind;
The five types of contempt:
Showing disrespect for the Buddhas or Dharma,
Hating friends of the world,
Spiritual leaders, members of the Sangha,
And deceiving those who trust me;
And the five longings:
Being infatuated with sights, sounds, fragrances,
Tastes, and tactile or physical sensations —
Restraining from these are the twenty-five modes of tamed behavior.
I shall safeguard, correctly and well, against these root downfalls
And faulty actions spoken of in *The Tantra of Kalachakra*.

Forsaking the four root destructive actions, likewise liquor and faulty
    behavior,
Committing myself whole-heartedly to a holy protecting guru,
Serving and treating respectfully Dharma friends,
Cultivating the ten constructive acts,
Avoiding the causes for forsaking mahayana,
Belittling it or treading on objects worthy of respect —
I shall honor these further practices to bond me closely.

Relying on an unqualified mudra partner,
Sitting in union devoid of the three recognitions,
Showing confidential objects to an unsuitable vessel,
Fighting or arguing when offering tsog,
Giving false answers to sincerely asked questions,
Staying more than a week in a shravaka's home,
Boasting that I am a yogi, although I am not,
Teaching the sacred Dharma to those with no faith,
Improperly engaging in mandala-rites, such as without a retreat,
Transgressing pratimoksha or bodhisattva trainings when there
    is no need,
Acting counter to the teachings of *Fifty Stanzas on the Guru* —
These are the secondary tantric heavy actions,
I shall safeguard against them in accord with the rules.

I shall not look down on left-handed behavior,
I shall offer tsog, reject sitting in union with an unqualified partner,
While in union, never be parted from a correct view,
Relentlessly aspire to the path of desire,
Not forsake the two kinds of mudra,
Exert effort mainly on the outer and inner methods,
Never release my subtle jasmine drops,
Commit myself to chaste behavior,
And abandon nausea when imbibing bodhichitta.

[B3]

I shall never transgress, even in dreams,
The most minor rule of the pure moral trainings
Of the pratimoksha, bodhisattva or tantric vows.
I shall practice according to Buddha's words.

As Buddha intended, I shall uphold the complete sacred Dharma
Of the scriptures and realizations gathered in
The three sutra vehicles and four tantra sets.
I shall liberate all beings by means that suit each.

[C1]

Just as those in the sage's clan, including Surya,
Attained deep discriminating awareness from this,
So may all beings throughout the three planes of existence
Likewise evolve through Kalachakra's kindness.

Just as the vajra of my enlightening mind shall remain
In infinite lands to liberate all beings,
So may these beings themselves, through the force of Kalachakra,
Do likewise and remain throughout the three realms.

May those persons who, through demonic friends,
Continually stray in the darkness of untruth and fall from the path,
Attain this spiritual path of the mind and, in not too long,
Arrive at the house of vajra-gems.

Through the force of the positive potential derived from this
And the power of Vajradhara, may I never transgress,
Throughout all my lives, the limits of my precepts.
May I complete the stages of the twofold path.

In brief, may I be born in Shambhala, the storehouse of gems,
And in as quick a time as the amount of ennobling,
Constructive potential I have gathered, for example by this,
Complete there the stages of this peerless path.

May I make full use of the glory of Dharma, never being bereft
Of perfect gurus throughout all my lives,
And by achieving in full the talents of all the stages and paths,
May I quickly attain Vajradhara-enlightenment.

[C2]

May the bodhisattvas dwelling above
In directions totaling the number of demons,
Utterly terrifying the would-be divine;

And the wrathful kings and queens dwelling either in or parted
From the main directions in the human world;
And the hooded naga lords beneath the earth,
Binding up, at their appropriate time,
Hordes of evil spirits and anything destructive,
Each deal with whatever is inauspicious
At their specific times during the day and night,
And provide the world with complete protection.

[OPTIONAL, BETWEEN C1 AND C2]

By the force of the vastly expanding ocean
Of my bountiful store of constructive potential
Which has come from the continuous gathering
Into the lake of my mind
Of a stainless stream of water of meditating,
Repeating mantras and making offerings
That flows from the snowy mountain
Of my pure and exceptional resolve like this,
Combined furthermore by my mind into one
With my entire store of constructive potential
Gathered throughout the three times,
May I be cared for, in life after life, by spiritual masters
Of the superlative vehicle as holy guiding lights.

By learning, from the guidelines they happily impart,
The methods gathered together in the three vehicles' Dharma,
And putting their meaningful points into practice,
May I mature my mind-stream with their paths shared in common.

By receiving the seven purifying empowerments,
May I soundly establish potentials for the seven levels of mind,
Cleanse myself of the seven stains, such as those on my elements,
And gain the power to actualize the first stage yogas and common
    attainments.

Through the four worldly and transcendent supreme empowerments,
May I plant the seeds for the four Buddha-bodies, the four vajra-features,
And acquire the power to study, explain and meditate on
The four branches approximating and actualizing the second stage.

May I sit majestically in the supreme palace of vajrayana, exquisite
    beyond measure,
On a throne of four purifying empowerments,
With a footstool of non-declining bonds and vows,
As an emperor with a wheel of authority over the two stages' measures.

Through cleansing out, then purifying myself
For an enlightening body, speech, mind and deep awareness,
And through the yoga of meditating that the six family-figures
[Are at my chakras] and [various syllables are] on my six limbs,
Then with a forceful blaze of lights from vajras
Arranged at particular spots in my body,
May I burn away demonic forces and interference.

From generating in the middle of the sphere of space
Four element discs, then merging them as one,
May I actualize a vajra-fence with five layers of thickness,
A three-layered one, a towering mansion, as well as the seats.

With stable absorbed concentration on myself in the center of these
As a glorious Vajra-vega, powerful lord of the forceful ones,
And by emanating out through all of my orifice-gates
A host of sixty spiritual guards, may I annihilate
Outer and inner demonic forces and interference.

By realizing, through the motions of emanating forth and gathering
    back in,
A bountiful field for merit pervading the entire sphere of space,
Then, as preparation, building up bountiful stores in accord with
    ritual procedures,
May I finish amassing great waves of bountiful stores.

Having accustomed myself to the pride of dharma-kaya
At the end of dissolving my half dozen elements like the stages of death,
May I reach the endpoint of absorbed concentration
    on the four gateways to total liberation,
Which herald enlightenment in the very moment.

By meditating on space, wind, fire, water and earth discs, as well as
    Mount Meru,
May I realize the abiding state of vajra-body
With features such as chakras at my crown and mid-brow,
My throat, heart, navel and pubic region.

By meditating being on top of a lotus, moon, sun
And Rahu and Kalagni discs, together with a tent made of vajras,
May I block the hosts of winds of my right and left channels
So they enter my conch one through supreme vajra-yoga.

By the force of meditating on a palace within the vajra-tent,
Exquisite beyond measure, imbued with the light of stainless gems,
May I purify fully a field where I shall become a Buddha
And remove obscuration from my body supported there.

By meditating on a moon and sun with vowels and consonants,
And two syllables of wind and mind,
All combining into one as a syllable *HAM*,
May I develop greatly blissful awareness
From gathering together in my central channel
My white and red sources and subtle wind and mind.

By the force of meditating that I arise from this with an enlightening body
Of a Kalachakra, endowed with the supreme of all aspects,
With a nature of greatly blissful awareness and complete in all parts,
Together with my lady of awareness and the deities of my great bliss circle,
May this become a cause to develop the supreme complete stages
Of mahamudra devoid-form and its being filled with the taste
Of unchanging, co-arising blissful awareness,
Which directly derive respectively from
The mudras with an aspect and lacking in one.

By meditating on the approximating branch, the supreme
    victorious mandala,
Which heralds enlightenment through its five aspects,
And, in which, out of seeds from myself, the father,
Absorbed in union with the mother,
I generate in her womb
A supreme circle of complete deities
And then settle them soundly, each at their spot,
May I cleanse my aggregate factors and elemental sources,
Cognitive sensors as well as their objects,
My functional parts and also their actions,
So that I may develop the supreme realizations of the paths of the mind.

By meditating on the nearly actualizing branch, the supreme
    victorious actions,
With its enlightenment through twenty aspects,
Namely the five-fold arousing, by tunes
Of divine maidens' melodious songs,
Of myself as Bhagavan Vajrin,
Together with my ladies of awareness,
All standing on the lotus of my great bliss chakra,
Where, through the force of having melted
With the fires of tummo at my navel,
We had taken the form of drops
Of greatly blissful awareness;
And likewise the five-fold arising; the five forceful ones;
And their hooking in [beings for deep awareness],
Merging, binding, pleasing and making them of equal taste
With the circle of those to bond me closely, which also make five;
And also with its conferring of empowerment,
Application of seals,
And mindfulness of the purifications,
May I manifest all their significance.

May I manifest the supreme actualizing branch, the yoga of the drop,
By imagining what represents the four levels
Of joyful awareness in emerging order,
Which come from consecrating our private place and space,

Absorbing in union,
And then rousing my downward voiding wind
To make the flames of my tummo blaze upwards
Through the pathway of my central channel
So that the coursing of my right and left energy-winds stop
And my bodhichitta, melting from the *HAM* at the crown of my head,
Descends in stages.

May I reach the endpoint of the greatly actualized branch, the subtle yoga,
With its four levels of joyful awareness that stabilize from below,
Rising upwards once more in the same order in which they came;
And also a web of emanated illusions which heralds enlightenment.

In short, may I reach the endpoint of my efforts
To meditate, in four sessions, on the supreme stage of generation,
The waters to cleanse me of making
Everything appear in its ordinary manner
And implying [it actually exists in that way],
The pathway of mind that ripens giving rise
To the complete stage's being complete,
And which purifies the outer and inner bases for purification.

By exerting myself, in addition, in repeating mantras,
Performing fire pujas and presenting offerings,
May I ripen infinite beings through being unimpeded
In realizing the actual attainment of the ultimate attainment —
To abide in Akanishta, the Realm Beneath Nothing.

May I accustom myself to the six-branch practice —
The yogas constructive for the start:
Individual collecting and constancy of mind;
Those constructive for the middle:
The paths of breath-control and holding;
And those constructive for the end:
Subsequent mindfulness and absorbed concentration.

With a manner of looking in which my eyes
Are partially closed and turned up
So that I feel they are penetrating the very core
Of the upper end of my central channel
Between the corners of my eyes,
May I fixate my mind single-pointedly at this spot,
Without mental dullness or flightiness of mind.

As a non-deceptive sign that resulting from this
The hosts of winds in my right and left channels
Have gathered into this spot in my central channel,
May I manifest the four night signs
That are like smoke, a mirage, flaring sparks in the sky
And a butter-lamp flame.

By meditating further, as before, with this manner of looking
At the space that is free of moisture-bearing clouds,
May I complete these [four] with the six further signs
Of blazing, then moon, sun, Rahu, lightning and a drop.

Through constancy of mind with which devoid-forms
Gather in stages at my body-drop's site
And which stays single-pointedly aimed at these forms, for as long
    as I wish,
May I induce from this a blissful sense of physical and mental fitness.

From the force of accustoming myself
Single-pointedly with these first two yogas,
Which actualize devoid-forms in this manner
And then stabilize whatever I have actualized,
May I achieve the power of my words coming true
And the five types of advanced awareness.

By accustoming myself to the breath-control practice
Of vajra-repetition, spontaneously accomplishing all,
In which my winds, indivisible from mantra,
Course through the pathway of my Rahu channel,

And to the breath-control practice of possessing a vase,
In which my upper and lower energy-winds
Are stopped at my navel,
May I have arise the distinguished signs
Of all hosts of my winds entering the center
Of my emanation chakra and abiding there slightly,
And thus manifest melodious sounds of the bodhisattvas' praise.

Through the yoga of holding my mind immobile and firm
In the center of my pair of life and downward energy-winds
Mixed into one at the hubs of my half dozen chakras,
May I then, at the end of enhancing four levels of joyful awareness
That fall from above and stabilize from below,
Arise in a devoid-form body on the face of my mind
And cause hordes of demonic forces of untimely death to decline.

Having well attained the force of all my devoid-forms
And vital winds being under control,
May I then, from a great co-arising blissful awareness
Induced by the blazing once more of the flames of my tummo,
Actually arise in the body of a devoid-form father and mother, joined
    in union,
And diffuse rays of light of assorted colors
Out the holes of the pores of my skin.

Joined in union with a mahamudra devoid-form partner like this,
May I meditate on great and unchanging blissful awareness,
Well induced by this mudra's own power,
And joined with voidness.

By the force of stacking my white and red sources
To the count of twenty-one thousand six hundred
Up and down through the path of my central channel,
May the elements of my corporeal matter
Be consumed like iron by mercury.

With twenty-one thousand six hundred moments
Of unchanging greatly blissful awareness that realize voidness,
May I stop the same number of winds of my karma
And cleanse myself quickly of all propensities for obscuration
And thereby attain the enlightening bodies of a triumphant Buddha.

May I actualize with ease, and without any hindrance,
These points to which I aspire like this,
And thus become a superior ship-captain
For freeing all beings, through this consummate path,
To the Buddhas' magnificent isle of jewels.

In brief, may I be born in Shambhala, the storehouse of gems,
And in as quick a time as the amount of ennobling,
Constructive potential I have gathered, for example by this,
Complete there the stages of this peerless path.

———————•◆•———————

If reciting six times each day in the manner of three times each morning
and three times each evening, recite the following sequence:

    [A] three times, omitting all [A-X] sections for the second and
         third repetitions,
    [B] three times, omitting all [B-X] sections for the second and
         third repetitions,
    [C] one time.